Home Remedies
For Asthma
And Bronchitis

Home Remedies
For Asthma
And Bronchitis

By Monica Sidoine,
S.N.H.S. Dip. Herbalism

DISCLAIMER

This book is to serve as an informational guide for use in the home. The remedies and procedures contained in this book are meant to supplement and are not intended to be a substitute for professional medical care. Please seek a qualified medical practitioner for all ailments. The author nor distributors takes no responsibility for customers choosing to treat themselves. Your use of this information is at your own risk.

ISBN - 13: 978-1533535733
ISBN - 10: 1533535736

Proof Read by Jasmine Ned Anunda

Printed By Create Space Publishing
United States of America

ACKNOWLEDGMENTS

I would like to thank all those who have contributed in one way or another to the completion of HOME REMEDIES FOR ASTHMA AND BRONCHITIS.

I thank God for giving me the vision, wisdom and good health to write this book. For all he has done and will continue to do in my life.

For the many prayer warriors who interceded on behalf of this project and also their moral support.

I thank my daughter Jasmine Ned Anunda for proof reading.

Thank you all.

Monica Sidoine.

PREFACE

The procedures in this Book was designed to be as simple as possible so that anyone will be able to follow them. Most of the items used are local things which you would either have at home, in your kitchen garden or can be easily purchased from the local market or health store for a very low cost.

TABLE OF CONTENTS

ASTHMA

Asthma is a disease of the respiratory system, sometimes caused by allergies.

Extrinsic, or Allergic asthma, is more common and typically develops in childhood. Approximately 70%-80% of children with asthma also have documented allergies. Typically, there is a family history of allergies. Additionally, other allergic conditions, such as nasal allergies or eczema, are often also present. Allergic asthma often goes into remission in early adulthood. However, in many cases, the asthma reappears later.

Intrinsic or Nonallergic asthma represents a small amount of all cases. It usually develops after the age of 30 and is not typically associated with allergies. Women are more frequently affected and many cases seem to follow a respiratory tract infection. The condition can be difficult to treat and symptoms are often chronic and year-round.

Symptoms including coughing, sudden difficulty in breathing and a tight feeling in the chest, a wheezing or whistling sound while breathing, congested chest, feeling tired while doing any physical activity, frequent cold and cough and uneasiness in sleeping.

Some causes of asthma attacks are dust, smoke, chemicals, stress, tension, depression, fear, changes in the temperature, low blood sugar, laughing, allergies, tobacco, environmental factors like air pollution, obesity, genetics, lung infection during childhood, premature birth, exercise, heartburn, certain foods like fish, soy, eggs, peanuts, etc.

NATURAL REMEDIES

- Chop and boil a 1ft piece of tamarind bark in 3 glasses of water for 10 minutes.
  Adults 1 cup after every meal and at bedtime, children ½ cup 4 times daily after meals and at bedtime, babies 2 teaspoons 4 times daily after meals and at bedtime.

- Boil 1oz of licorice root in 1 liter of water for 15 minutes. Add the juice of ½ a lime and a 1" piece of crushed ginger to it.
  Drink 1 cup three times daily.

- Blend 2 garlic cloves with 2 cups of boiling water until thoroughly blended. Add a pinch of salt and a drop of eucalyptus oil.
  The 1st cupful should be drunk rapidly.
  In some persons the hot garlic water may cause vomiting which helps to loosen the bronchial secretions, makes coughing successful and helps to improve breathing. The 2nd cup should be taken promptly after vomiting.

- Blend four cloves of garlic in a cup of lukewarm water until thoroughly blended.
  Drink it rapidly.
  Most persons will have nausea and vomiting after drinking it which assists greatly in loosening bronchial secretions, makes coughing successful and helps to improve breathing. Make a second cup of the garlic water, blending only one clove of garlic in a cup of cold water or tomato juice. Sip and drink promptly after the vomiting has entirely stopped.

- Boil 6 cloves in half a glass of water. Add a tablespoon of honey. Take it twice daily.

- Boil 1 tablespoon of fenugreek seeds in a cup of water. Add 1 teaspoon each of ginger juice and honey in it.
  Drink it twice daily.

- Crush 8 cloves of garlic and boil it in 1 cup of milk till it reduces to ½ cup.
  Take it at bedtime.

- Mix one teaspoon honey and ¼ teaspoon cinnamon powder.
  Take it twice daily.

- Mix 1 teaspoon honey in a cup of hot water.
  Take it in small sips just before bedtime.

- Take 1 tablespoon of sunflower or corn oil just before bedtime.

- Boil 1oz of ginger in 1 liter of water for 15 minutes.
  Drink 1 cup three times daily.

- Boil 1 grapefruit skin in 1 ½ gallons of water for 30 minutes.
  Take 2 tablespoons several times a day.

- **Eucalyptus Syrup:**
  Boil 1oz of dried eucalyptus leaves in 2 cups of water for 10 minutes. Steep for 20 minutes. Strain and add 11oz of honey. Bottle.
  Take 1 teaspoon 3 times daily.

- Steep 1oz of chamomile in 1 liter of boiling water for 20 minutes.
  Take 6oz 3 times daily.

- Steep 1oz of anise in 1 liter of boiling water for 30 minutes.
  Drink 1 cup 4 times daily.

- Steep 1oz of peppermint in 1 liter of boiling water for 30 minutes.
  Drink 1 cup 4 times daily.

- Add 1 tablespoon of lemon juice in 1 cup of hot water.
  Drink 1 cup every 2 hours.

- Steep 1 teaspoon of cayenne to 1 cup of boiling water for 20 minutes.
  Take 3½ teaspoons or 1-2 capsules 3 times daily.

  N.B. Very excessive use can damage the kidneys.

- Using either one of the following combinations: Eucalyptus and thyme, or Marjoram, thyme and savory. Put 1oz of the herbs in 2 pints of boiling water and steep for 20 minutes.
  Take 1 cup three times daily.

- Steep 1oz of lemon leaves in 1 liter of boiling water for 20 minutes. It can be sweetened with honey.
  Drink 4 cups daily.

- Steep 1oz of parsley leaves in 1 liter of boiling water for 20 minutes.
  Drink 3 cups daily.

- Mix 1 teaspoon of ground ginger in 1 ½ cups of water.
  Take 1 tablespoon at bedtime.

- Stir ½ teaspoon powdered turmeric in 1 cup of hot milk, add a pinch of salt, ginger or cayenne.
  Drink 1 cup 3 times daily.

- Mix equal quantities of ginger juice, pomegranate juice and honey.
  Consume 1 tablespoon three times a day.

- Combine 1 teaspoon each of onion and ginger juice along with 1 tablespoon of honey.
  Take it twice daily.

- Add 1 tablespoon each of olive oil and honey to a glass of warm milk.
  Drink it along with 4 raw garlic cloves, before having breakfast.

- Combine 1 tablespoon each of ginger juice and of honey along with 2 tablespoons of dried fenugreek seeds. Soak it overnight. Take it every morning.

- Drink Sugar cane juice.

- Boil 9oz of peeled sugarcane to 1 liter of water for 30 minutes. Take 1 cup 4 times daily.

- Drink lots of water.

- Soak 3 dried figs in a cup of water overnight.
  In the morning, eat the soaked figs and drink the fig water on an empty stomach.
  Do this treatment for a few months.

- Blend a radish and strain to get the juice. Mix it with some honey and lemon juice.
  Consume it.

- Extract the juice of bitter gourd. Make a paste of basil and honey. Add it to the bitter gourd juice mixing it well.

- Eat raw ginger mixed with salt.

- Eat lots of raw garlic and onions.

- Eat lots of strawberries, blueberries, papaya and oranges.

- Crush some gooseberries and add some honey to it.
  Consume it daily.

- Make small herb pillows with fresh rosemary and have it close when sleeping to help with breathing.

- Put a few drops of eucalyptus oil on a paper towel or handkerchief.
  Keep it by your head when sleeping so that you can breathe in the aroma.

- Do deep breathing exercises. Inhaling through the nose and exhaling through the mouth.

- Warm some mustard oil with a little camphor.
  Gently rub it on the chest and upper back and massage.
  Do it several times a day until the symptoms decrease.

- Put 2 to 3 drops of eucalyptus oil in a pan of boiling water.
  Use it as a steam inhalation.
  See the Hydrotherapy Section.

- Steep 1oz chamomile in 1 liter of boiling water for 30 minutes.
  Use it as a steam inhalation.
  See the Hydrotherapy Section.

- Boil one aloe leaf in a pan of water.
  Use it as a steam inhalation.
  See the Hydrotherapy Section.

- Boil 3 potatoes in a pan of water.
  Use it as a steam inhalation.
  See the Hydrotherapy Section.

- Boil 2 tablespoons of thyme in 1 liter of water for 30 minutes.
  Use it as a steam inhalation.
  See the Hydrotherapy Section.

- **GARLIC HAND AND FOOT BATH**

  Procedure:
  1. Crush 5 garlic cloves and pour ¾ gallons of boiling water over it. Cover and steep for half day.
  2. Heat it and then strain. Use it as a hand and foot bath together for 30 minutes daily.
  3. Put the feet and hands in the hot bath for 3 minutes and then in the cold bath for 1 minute ending with the cold bath. Repeat 7 times.

Health Tips

- Avoid dairy products.

- Avoid foods that are very cold.

- Avoid fried foods.

- Avoid fish.

- Avoid food additives.

- Avoid alcohol.

- Avoid caffeine and smoking.

- Try to get as much fresh air as possible.

BRONCHITIS

Bronchitis is an inflammation of the mucous membrane in the airways bronchial tubes of the lungs.

Acute bronchitis, also known as a chest cold, is short term inflammation of the bronchi of the lungs.

The most common symptom is a cough. Other symptoms include coughing up mucus, wheezing, shortness of breath, fever, and chest discomfort.

The infection may last from a few to ten days. The cough may persist for several weeks afterwards with the total duration of symptoms usually around three weeks. Some have symptoms for up to six weeks.

Risk factors include exposure to tobacco smoke, dust, and other air pollution. A small number of cases are due to high levels of air pollution or bacteria.

Chronic bronchitis is defined as a productive cough that lasts for three months or more per year for at least two years. Most people with chronic bronchitis have chronic obstructive pulmonary disease (COPD).

Tobacco smoking is the most common cause, with a number of other factors such as air pollution and genetics playing a smaller role.

Symptoms of chronic bronchitis may include wheezing and shortness of breath, especially upon exertion and low oxygen saturations. The cough is often worse soon after awakening and the sputum produced may have a yellow or green color and may be streaked with specks of blood.

Treatments include quitting smoking, vaccinations, rehabilitation, and often inhaled bronchodilators and steroids. Some people may benefit from long-term oxygen therapy or lung transplantation.

This respiratory disease is primarily caused by the bacteria or viruses which irritate the bronchial tubes. Some other causes of this ailment are as follows: - allergy, infections, cough and cold, changes in the atmosphere, smoking, dusty air or fog and pollution.

Some common signs and symptoms are breathing problems, severe coughing, soreness in the chest, sore throat, fatigue, watery eyes, chest pain or tightening of chest, coughing with mucous, fever, muscle ache and nasal congestion.

NATURAL REMEDIES

- Steep 1 teaspoon of cayenne powder in 1 cup of boiling water for 20 minutes.
  Take it by ½ fluid oz. doses or 2 capsules 3 times daily.

  N.B. Very excessive use can damage the kidneys.

- **Turnip syrup:** Put 2lbs of peeled sliced turnips on a flat dish. Cover it with 1lb of brown sugar. Leave it to rest for 12 hours. Strain and put the liquid in a bottle.
  Take 2 tablespoons daily.

- Slice 1 onion in a bowl and cover it with honey. Leave it overnight. Remove the onion slices.
  Take 1 teaspoon of honey four times daily.

- Add 1 teaspoon of honey to hot lemon drink.
  Drink it first thing in the morning and during the day.

- Add 1 teaspoon of grated lemon rind to 1 cup of boiling water. Steep it for 10 minutes.
  Drink it daily.

- Boil 6 bay leaves in 1 liter of water for 4 minutes. Steep for 5 minutes. It can be sweetened with honey.
  Drink 1 cup 4 times daily.

- Boil 1oz of licorice root in 1 liter of water for 15 minutes.
  Drink 1 cup twice daily.

- Boil 1oz thyme in 1 liter of water for 10 minutes. Steep for 10 minutes.
  Drink I cup 4 times daily.

- Add 1 teaspoon of turmeric powder in a glass of milk. Stir it well and bring to a boil.
  Drink it hot 3 times daily on an empty stomach.

- Boil 2 tablespoons of eucalyptus leaves in 1 liter of water for 4 minutes. Steep for 5 minutes. It can be sweetened with honey.
  Drink 1 cup 4 times daily.

- Add 3 crushed garlic cloves in a glass of milk. Bring it to a boil.
  Drink it warm just before bedtime.

- Boil 2 tablespoons of rosemary in 1 liter of water for 4 minutes. Steep for 5 minutes. It can be sweetened with honey.
  Drink 1 cup 4 times daily.

- Boil 5 cloves and 6 eucalyptus leaves in 1 pint of water for 3 minutes. Steep for 5 minutes. Strain and add the juice of ½ of a lemon to it.
  Drink ½ cup 4 times daily.

- Combine powdered ginger, cloves, and cinnamon together. Add half teaspoon of the mixture in a glass of hot water. Stir it very well.
  Drink it twice daily for a few days.

- Combine 1 teaspoon each of honey, ground flaxseed and sesame seeds. Add a pinch of salt to it.
  Take it daily at bedtime.

- Mix ½ teaspoon of dry sesame seeds powder in 2 tablespoons of water.
  Take it daily.

- Boil 9oz of peeled sugarcane to 1 liter of water for 20 minutes.
  Drink 1 cup 4 times daily.

- Grind half teaspoon of almonds and stir it in a glass of orange juice.
  Drink it at night.

- Drink sugar cane juice daily.

- Take 1 teaspoon of raw onion juice on an empty stomach every morning.

- Blend 5 spinach leaves in a glass of water. Add ½ tablespoon honey to it and drink it.

- Have vegetable and fruit juices.

- Drink at least 10 glasses of water daily.

- Eat lots of raw onions and garlic, watercress, radishes, okra and almonds.

- Apply a few drops of oregano oil under the tongue.
  Do it once daily.

- Put 1 teaspoon salt into 2 glasses of hot water, stir until it is melted. The water temperature should be to as hot as can be tolerated for drinking.
  Gargle till all 2 glasses is used up. It is best done after meals.

- Add 1 teaspoon of lemon juice in a cup of warm water. Stir it well and gargle with it.

- Combine 10 drops each of rosemary oil, thyme, peppermint and eucalyptus oil. Add ¼ cup of olive oil or coconut oil to it. Gently massage it on the chest and throat.

- Combine 2 teaspoons olive or coconut oil and 1 teaspoon thyme oil. Gently massage the chest and throat.

- Add 3 drops of peppermint or eucalyptus essential oil to 1 teaspoon of almond or coconut oil. Massage your throat and chest with it. Place a warm towel over the affected area.

- Put 1lb of Epsom salt in warm bath water. Soak in it for half an hour nightly just before bedtime. Do it twice daily if you have chronic bronchitis.

- **Steam inhalation**- 3 drops of eucalyptus oil to a bowl of hot water, inhale for 5 minutes. 3-4 times daily. Put a few drops on a handkerchief and inhale. Massage the abdomen and upper part of the body excluding the head and arms 3 times daily with 2oz of coconut oil and 15 drops of eucalyptus oil.

- **Mustard Poultice:** Mix 1 tablespoon of dry mustard to 4 tablespoons of wheat flour for an adult, 1 tablespoon mustard to 8 tablespoons flour for a child, 1 tablespoon mustard to 12 tablespoons flour for an infant. Add enough lukewarm water to make a thin paste. Spread it on a cloth and fold over. Apply some olive oil over the chest. Place a thin cotton cloth over the effected part. Put on the poultice, then a large piece of plastic to cover it and a towel. A warm towel or hot water bottle can be applied over this to increase the heat. Remove it earlier if it is burning, stinging, or the skin has become well reddened. Wipe the area with a cloth or paper tissue dipped in vegetable oil to remove the mustard. Cover the area with a warm blanket and leave on overnight. Leave it on for 20 minutes.

- Soak bay leaves in hot water. Apply it as a poultice on the chest. Cover the chest with a towel. Rewarm it whenever it cools down.

- Apply a flaxseed poultice to the chest and the back.
  Mix 1 tablespoon of coconut oil with 5 drops of eucalyptus oil and 2 drops of oregano oil. Use this to rub into the chest and the back after removing the poultice.

  Flaxseed Poultice: Grind 2 tablespoons of flaxseed, mix it with 2 cups of water. Stir briskly with a wooden spoon. Spread the mixture on a piece of damp cloth, over a paper towel or directly on the skin. Cover with a larger piece of plastic, hold in place with a strip of cloth or a bandage. Leave it on for 30 minutes to 8 hours or overnight. Remove it, wash the area with a washcloth, and then give a cold mitten friction, dry thoroughly.

- Vaporize the room during the day and at least one hour before bedtime. Mix 1 pint of warm water with 15 drops of tea tree oil and 5 drops of lavender essential oil or 15 drops of eucalyptus oil and 5 drops of oregano oil. Shake it well before using.

Health Tips

- Try to get adequate rest daily.

- Avoid alcohol and smoking.

- Avoid dairy products, white flour products and sugary items.

- Avoid contact with scented candles, air fresheners, etc.

- Avoid air pollutants.

- Wash and rinse hands and face as often as possible.

HYDROTHERAPY TREATMENT

STEAM INHALATION

Effects:

1. Relieves nasal and lung congestions.

2. Relieves coughs.

3. Secretions are loosen and it is easier to expectorate.

4. Blood flow is increased to the throat and lungs.

5. Relieves sinus headaches.

Contraindications:

1. Persons suffering with congestive heart failure.

2. Persons suffering with asthma.

Items needed:

Basin with boiling water
Umbrella and sheet
Bedside stand and chair
A few drops of wintergreen or eucalyptus oil,
or 1 teaspoon Vicks VapoRub, or 2 tablespoons of herbs.

Procedure:

1. Fill a face basin with boiling water and add medication or herb if desired.

2. Put it on a table or bedside stand. Sit on a chair and open an umbrella over the head then cover with a sheet to form a tent over the head and basin. Instead of the umbrella and sheet, a large thick towel can be used to cover the head and basin.

3. Inhale the steam for 30 to 60 minutes 2 – 3 times daily.

4. Dry the face and any other moist areas of the body.

5. Rest for half an hour.

Other Book Titles by the Same Author

Can be viewed at this link:
http://www.amazon.com/author/monicasidoine

Home Remedies For Cancer

Home Remedies For Losing Weight

Home Remedies For Blood Pressure and Diabetes

Home Remedies For Headaches and Insomnia

Home Remedies For Sinusitis and Tonsillitis

Home Remedies For Constipation and Diarrhea

Home Remedies For Dehydration and Vomiting

Home Remedies For Pneumonia and Tuberculosis

Home Remedies For Stress, Depression and Anxiety

NOTES

NOTES

NOTES